Smoothies for Weight Loss

Top 27 delicious smoothies that burn fat, keep you slim, energetic and healthy

By Linda April

Disclaimer

All the material contained in this book is provided for educational and informational purposes only. No responsibility can be taken for any results or outcomes resulting from the use of this material.

While every attempt has been made to provide information that is both accurate and effective, the author does not assume any responsibility for the accuracy or use/misuse of this information.

Some examples of past results are used in this publication; they are intended to be for example purposes only and do not guarantee you will get the same results. Your results may differ and your results from the use of this information will depend on you, your skills and effort, and other different unpredictable factors.

Acknowledgements

Couple of years back, I was suffering from a health condition in which I was continuously gaining my body weight. All of my friends used to tease me and often they call me a FAT LADY. It was really embarrassing and I used to avoid going outside and prefer to stay at home.

Well I spent almost 1000s of dollars in the gym but was of no use.

Later, I met Jennifer (a professional nutritionist), who laughed at my condition and told me that exercise won't burn the stored fat in a short period of time. I need to try something else!

She gave me a list of few recipes and asked me to try those early in the morning, on an unfilled stomach. She didn't even charge anything for those recipes as she was going through the same condition.

I tried those drinks early in the morning and it really worked well. I managed to lose approximately 60 pounds in just 30 days. It was simply unbelievable but it's real. It's all natural and you just need to consume lots of fresh fruits or vegetables.

These recipes are so delicious and mouth-tempting that I couldn't stop myself sharing them.

Preface

You definitely need a strong willpower along with the correct way, if are you are planning for losing weight & getting the results you were looking for as smoothies are one of the finest ways to lose weight effectively. However, it's not that simple as everything just depends on your body condition & your desire to lose.

You would surely be able to lose those added pounds, if you include a lot of fresh fruits & vegetables in your daily diet as smoothies that come from fresh fruits and vegetables are generally very low in calories & include plenty of micro-nutrients which are essential for you to grow. Additionally, it helps keeping the natural fiber present in the foods.

You would be able to maintain your body weight & you can actually do miracles to your health if you drink smoothies that you get from fresh & organic fruits or vegetables every single day, preferably on an unfilled stomach.

You'll realize that you don't have to be an exercise "freak" in order to prevent your body from overweight, heart disease, diabetes & some types of cancer. Your energy level would rise and you would actually feel good.

Smoothies are just delicious & doable and you can prepare it in a very short period of time. When we say yes to health, we say no to harm.

In the subsequent of this e-book, I would share 27 delicious smoothies that burn Fat, keep you slim, energetic and healthy throughout the day.

Table of Contents

Chapter 1: Introduction

Natural products smoothies can be a simple approach to feed your body with fundamental supplements. The most ideal approach to know the careful fixings in your smoothie is to make them yourself. Everything you need is a blender, foods grown from the ground base, for example, water, milk or yogurt. Making your own smoothies can keep organic product from going to squander, while giving advantages that will keep you in good shape towards great wellbeing.

Why do as such numerous individuals devour sound smoothies all the time? I have my own reasons, however thought it would be fun and supportive for others to gather the majority of the more famous reasons into one spot. At first, I anticipated covering the main 10 reasons, yet once I got going I understood 10 wouldn't do equity to sound smoothies.

While a hefty portion of the reasons underneath are connected with a specific medical advantage, a few others made the rundown. Subsequent to perusing this I think you'll be persuaded that adding to the propensity for making solid smoothies once a day is a fabulous venture of your time and cash.

Green smoothies have numerous medical advantages, and can incorporate spinach, lettuce, kale, and collard greens; for the more propelled green smoothie consumer, you can likewise include parsley, dandelion greens, and watercress— truly, any verdant green veggie your sense of taste can deal with, and appreciate. Bananas, apples, pears, avocado, and mango are awesome allies in these refreshments.

Here's a brief prologue to the numerous focal points of drinking green smoothies once a day.

Chapter 2: Top 24 Health Benefits

Get your daily share of fruits and vegetables

Devouring the everyday suggestions of products of the soil can be a test. Mixing several servings of each into a smoothie guarantees you meet your body's day by day nourishing necessities. Green smoothies can be a decent approach to get children to "eat" their vegetables. You may need to begin with a higher extent of organic product versus vegetables (for instance, 70/30 rather than the standard 60/40) until they get used to the flavour.

Quick and Easy

Making your own supplement thick smoothie doesn't take the length of planning most dinners, giving you more opportunity for others things. Bringing a smoothie with you is an extra advantageous choice.

Kids love Smoothies

Getting your children to eat solid nourishments is not generally simple. Luckily, most children love the essence of a velvety smoothie actually sweetened by natural product or a decent sweetener like nectar, maple syrup, or stevia. You can even shroud veggies in your child's smoothies that they could never eat all alone.

Easy Weight Loss

There are various health improvement plans that advance supplanting a supper with a fluid beverage. Furnish your body with every one of the vitamins and minerals it needs by means of smoothies, cut out the weight picking up food from your eating routine, and watch the pounds soften away. Get thinner simpler than before and thin down the solid path with eating regimen smoothies.

Improves Digestion

No one I know needs to experience blockage or heartburn. Give your blender "a chance to bite" your nourishment and facilitate the weight on your digestive framework while you at the same time devour a lot of dietary fiber to guarantee fantastic processing. Green smoothies are anything but difficult to process. Since they're now mixed and condensed, smoothies are snappier to process. All things considered, your body no more needs to work so difficult to "separate" the nourishment keeping in mind the end goal to remove the supplements. Individuals who experience the ill effects of heartburn in the wake of eating a substantial supper will likewise advantage, as smoothies are filling yet light.

Delicious

Yes, eating sound and tasting incredible can go as an inseparable unit. With such a large number of formulas to look over, discovering one or all the more satisfying to your sense of taste is a breeze.

Detox

We're presented to and shelled by a great many man-made chemicals in today's reality, which leaves our body asking to detoxify. Offer your digestive framework a reprieve while including detoxifying fixings like dandelion greens and kale into your smoothies to help your body's detoxification forms.

Builds Muscles and Improves Athletic Performance

Give your body the supplements it needs to exceed expectations amid athletic rivalry, and recuperate and remake in the wake of working out. It's simpler for your body to retain and absorb the supplements in a smoothie rather than a dinner.

Vitamins and Minerals

There are six classes of natural products that contain an assortment of vitamins and minerals- - citrus, berries, tropical, drupes, pomes and melons. Citrus natural products, for example, grapefruit, oranges, tangerines and lemons, contain great measures of vitamin C, potassium and folate. Vitamin C helps your invulnerable framework and incorporates collagen that guides in the structure of your body. Potassium underpins your heart capacity and keeps up a typical circulatory strain, while folate advances solid cells. The berry class incorporates blueberries, strawberries, blackberries, raspberries, cranberries and grapes. They contain specific cancer prevention agents that diminishing aggravation and phytonutrients that battle ailment. Tropical organic products incorporate papaya, kiwi natural product, pineapple, avocado, coconut, pomegranates, bananas and mangoes. Regularly, these natural products are wellsprings of vitamin C, potassium, folate and manganese, which keeps your bones, glucose, thyroid organ and nerves solid. Regular drupes organic products are fruits, apricots, peaches and plums. They give beta carotene, potassium and vitamin C. Beta carotene helps your vision and safe framework work legitimately. Pomes natural products incorporate apples and pears, which contain vitamin C and potassium. The melon classification incorporates watermelon, melon, nectar dew and casaba, which all contain sufficient measures of vitamin C.

Fiber

Drinking organic product smoothies can offer you some assistance with reaching the suggested admission of fiber, which is 25 grams for ladies and 38 grams for men. One serving of natural product regularly contains two to four grams of fiber with blackberries, pears and apples having the most noteworthy centralization of five to seven grams for every serving. The dissolvable fiber found in organic product moderates processing and might control glucose and lower cholesterol.

Smoothie Base

Making your own smoothie implies you get the opportunity to pick a base of your loving. You can include water, dairy animals' milk, soy milk or yogurt to the natural product keeping in mind the end goal to include mass. The more advantageous choices would incorporate water, low-fat drain or low-fat yogurt, which will include flavor and supplements without countless. The water will give your body liquid that is essential for digestion system of nourishment and transportation of supplements. The low-fat dairy contains calcium and vitamin D, which offer your bones some assistance with staying solid.

Beauty

Think brilliant skin, hair, and nails. Supply your body with the vitamins and minerals it requires to develop more beneficial hair and make your skin sparkle.

Healthy Habit

By realizing what constitutes a sound smoothie, you'll additionally teach yourself on what contains a solid eating regimen. This will permit you to settle on better choices when the blender isn't around. You'll be more positive about your sustenance decisions. Green smoothies are an awesome approach to eat your veggies without acknowledging it. Albeit the vast majority like organic product, numerous experience difficulty getting their day by day necessity of veggies. When you make a green smoothie, the essence of the greens is covered up by the essence of the organic product, so you don't notice the veggies are there.

Strengthens your Immune System

Becoming ill is unpleasant. Lessen the quantity of times you become ill (if by any means) and lesson the seriousness by enabling your safe framework.

Deeper Sleep

Consuming so as to enhance your wellbeing sound smoothies quite often brings about better rest during the evening.

Meal Flexibility

You can expend a smoothie at any feast, not simply breakfast. No time for lunch, snatch or make a speedy smoothie. Green smoothies are low in calories yet extremely filling. Since they contain high measures of water and fiber, they'll make you feel as though you just ate a full supper. In case you're attempting to get fit, green smoothies will battle yearning and desires while offering the pounds some assistance with melting off simpler.

Rich in Ingredients

The quantity of solid fixings accessible for smoothies is for all intents and purposes boundless. After your essential leafy foods, you can include a variety of the different flavours, herbs, super foods, and other wellbeing sustenance. The potential outcomes and blends are inestimable.

Energy

Supply your body with the right fuel for more vitality in the short and long haul. Green smoothies will give you an enduring wellspring of vitality. Organic products are a decent wellspring of vitality, however eaten alone will just give short blasts of vitality (they contain loads of sugars, which are immediately metabolized). Due to their high substance of veggies, green smoothies have adjusted sugar content.

Empowerment

Take control of your wellbeing through straightforward and delightful solid smoothies.

Reduce Cravings

We as a whole hunger for desserts and unfortunate nourishments every now and then. Diminish those desires, or even better, supplant what you would ordinarily binge spend on with a solid option.

Brain Boost

Give your mind every one of the vitamins and supplements it needs to enhance your mental clarity, centre, and memory. Say farewell to cerebrum haze.

Happiness

Experience a restored feeling of quiet and prosperity that great wellbeing prompts. Be in a decent temperament constantly.

Fun

Numerous individuals including myself observe making smoothies to be fairly pleasant. You can consider yourself a current chemist blending and coordinating different smoothie fixings.

Economical

Natively constructed green smoothies are modest. Purchasing smoothies at a juice bar can set you back as much as $6 a glass. At home, consolidating foods grown from the ground won't cost you more than a couple of pennies. Drinking a glass each day will furnish you with every one of the vitamins you require, a much less expensive (and more common) alternative than purchasing multivitamins.

Keeps you hydrated

Green smoothies will keep you hydrated. Albeit one ought to drink no less than eight glasses of water a day, specialists accept the vast majority don't drink even a large portion of that sum. One reason for that will be that numerous individuals just don't care for the essence of plain water. On the off chance that that portrays you, basically add more water to the blend as you set up your smoothie. You'll be drinking more fluids without seeing it.

Chapter 3: Recipes

Smoothie 1

Frozen Pineapple Smoothie

Total preparation & making time: 05 Minutes
Servings: 1

Nutrition Info (Estimated Amount Per Serving)

49.7 Calories
1 Calories from Fat
0.2 g Total Fat
0 g Saturated Fat
0 mg Cholesterol
10.3 mg Sodium
13.5 g Total Carbohydrate
2 g Dietary Fiber
8.8 g Sugars
0.8 g Protein

Ingredients:

- 1/2 cup pineapple, frozen
- 1/4 tsp. Stevia
- 1/2 cup ice cube
- 2 mint leaves, fresh
- 1/2 lemon
- 3/4 cup water

Directions:

1. Put pineapple together with the water & ice to a high speed blender.
2. Extract the juice from the lemon & add it to the blender along with stevia. Puree on high settings until smooth & creamy.
3. Garnish the mixture with mint leaves. Enjoy with 8 to 10 rice crackers.

Smoothie 2

Watermelon Smoothie

Total preparation & making time: 05 Minutes
Servings: 4

Nutrition Info (Estimated Amount Per Serving)

25.5 Calories
1 Calories from Fat
0.1 g Total Fat
0 g Saturated Fat
0 mg Cholesterol
6.2 mg Sodium
6.5 g Total Carbohydrate
0.3 g Dietary Fiber
4.8 g Sugars
0.6 g Protein

Ingredients:

1. 2 cups watermelon, cubed, seeded & freeze until firm
2. 1 can diet soda, preferably lemon-lime & chilled
3. 2 tbsp. lime juice, fresh
4. 1 cup ice cube, large size

Directions:

1. Place watermelon into a high speed blender and in the lime juice and process on high settings until smooth.
2. Add in the ice cubes, with blender still on, preferably one at a time and process again on high settings until smooth.
3. Add in the soda; whirl for couple of seconds to blend.
4. Serve immediately

Smoothie 3

Mouth-Tempting Watermelon Smoothie

Total preparation & making time: 10 Minutes
Servings: 1

Nutrition Info (Estimated Amount Per Serving)

94.2 Calories
3 Calories from Fat
0.4 g Total Fat
0 g Saturated Fat
0 mg Cholesterol
3 mg Sodium
24.6 g Total Carbohydrate
1.1 g Dietary Fiber
19 g Sugars
1.6 g Protein

Ingredients:

- 1 and 1/2 cups watermelon, seeded & cubed
- 1 tsp. Sugar, granulated
- Juice of 1 lime, fresh
- Mint sprig, fresh for garnish

Directions:

1. Add everything (except the mint sprig) to a high speed blender and blend on high settings until smooth & creamy.
2. Pour the watermelon mixture into a glass, preferably 12 oz. full with the ice cubes & garnish with fresh mint sprig.
3. Serve & enjoy!

Smoothie 4

Spinach Banana Smoothie

Total preparation & making time: 05 Minutes
Servings: 4

Nutrition Info (Estimated Amount Per Serving)

118.6 Calories
28 Calories from Fat
3.2 g Total Fat
1.9 g Saturated Fat
11.1 mg Cholesterol
87.4 mg Sodium
19.6 g Total Carbohydrate
2.9 g Dietary Fiber
11.5 g Sugars
5.3 g Protein

Ingredients:
- 1 banana, medium, frozen & sliced
- 6 oz. vanilla yogurt
- 4 cups Baby Spinach, raw
- Mint sprig, fresh
- Water or milk

Directions:
1. First of all you need to place spinach into a high speed blender and then

pour the yogurt over the spinach followed by the sliced banana.

2. Blend on high settings approximately a minute or two. To get the desired consistency, you may adjust the quantity of water; add more if seems too thick!

3. Garnish with fresh mint.

4. Serve & enjoy!

Smoothie 5

Strawberry Orange Smoothie

Total preparation & making time: 10 Minutes
Servings: 1

Nutrition Info (Estimated Amount Per Serving)

89.4 Calories
4 Calories from Fat
0.5 g Total Fat
0 g Saturated Fat
0 mg Cholesterol
5.7 mg Sodium
21.3 g Total Carbohydrate
1.7 g Dietary Fiber
16.8 g Sugars
1.4 g Protein

Ingredients:
- 1/2 cup strawberry, fresh & chopped
- 1/2 tsp. honey
- 1/2 cup ice cube
- 1/2 cup orange juice

Directions:
1. Add everything to a high speed blender and blend on high settings until smooth & creamy.

2. Pour the mixture to a tall glass, preferably chilled. Serve & enjoy!

Smoothie 6

Berry Watermelon Smoothie

Total preparation & making time: 10 Minutes
Servings: 4

Nutrition Info (Estimated Amount Per Serving)

141.6 Calories
5 Calories from Fat
0.6 g Total Fat
0.1 g Saturated Fat
0 mg Cholesterol
4.1 mg Sodium
35.6 g Total Carbohydrate
2.5 g Dietary Fiber
21.1 g Sugars
2.5 g Protein

Ingredients:
- 1 to 2 bananas, medium & frozen
- 1/4 watermelon
- 125 grams mixed berries, frozen or fresh
- 1/4 to 1/2 cup soy milk or rice milk
- Ice cubes, large (optional)
- Honey
- Cinnamon

Directions:

1. Add watermelon into a juicer, preferably on high settings.
2. To make a thick smoothie, you may add in the bananas accordingly.
3. Throw in the remaining ingredients, to taste.
4. Pour the mixture to four glasses. Serve & enjoy!

Smoothie 7

Blackberry Peach Smoothie

Total preparation & making time: 10 Minutes
Servings: 1

Nutrition Info (Estimated Amount Per Serving)

159.1 Calories
9 Calories from Fat
1 g Total Fat
0.2 g Saturated Fat
2.5 mg Cholesterol
75 mg Sodium
33.4 g Total Carbohydrate
5.5 g Dietary Fiber
21.8 g Sugars
7.2 g Protein

Ingredients:

- 1/3 cup blackberries, frozen
- 2 peaches, medium, peeled & quartered
- 1/2 cup skim milk or soymilk
- 3/4 cup ice cube
- honey to taste (optional)

Directions:

1. Add everything to your blender's container. Blend on high settings approximately 3 to 4 minutes, until ice is completely crushed and the mixture is smooth.
2. Taste & adjust the sweetness to your taste.

Smoothie 8

Orange Pineapple Smoothie

Total preparation & making time: 10 Minutes
Servings: 1

Nutrition Info (Estimated Amount Per Serving)

141.8 Calories
4 Calories from Fat
0.5 g Total Fat
0.1 g Saturated Fat
0 mg Cholesterol
5.5 mg Sodium
34.5 g Total Carbohydrate
1.9 g Dietary Fiber
23.9 g Sugars
1.8 g Protein

Ingredients:

- 1/2 banana, medium
- 1/4 cup pineapple juice
- 1/2 cup orange juice
- 1/4 to 1/2 tsp. gingerroot, fresh, peeled & grated
- 1/2 cup ice, crushed

Directions:

1. Add everything to a high speed blender and blend on high settings until smooth & creamy.
2. Pour the mixture to a tall glass. Serve & enjoy!

Smoothie 9

Strawberry Banana Smoothie

Total preparation & making time: 05 Minutes
Servings: 3

Nutrition Info (Estimated Amount Per Serving)

88.8 Calories
4 Calories from Fat
0.6 g Total Fat
0.2 g Saturated Fat
1 mg Cholesterol
14.8 mg Sodium
21.4 g Total Carbohydrate
2.7 g Dietary Fiber
12.2 g Sugars
1.8 g Protein

Ingredients:
- 8 strawberries, fresh
- 2 bananas, medium & frozen
- 1/4 cup milk, low-fat
- 2 cups ice, crushed

Directions:
1. Add everything to a high speed blender and blend on high settings

until smooth & creamy. Pour the mixture to glasses. Serve & enjoy!

Smoothie 10

Blackberry Banana Smoothie

Total preparation & making time: 05 Minutes
Servings: 1

Nutrition Info (Estimated Amount Per Serving)

233.1 Calories
10 Calories from Fat
1.2 g Total Fat
0.5 g Saturated Fat
4.9 mg Cholesterol
148.8 mg Sodium
46.7 g Total Carbohydrate
5.3 g Dietary Fiber
23.3 g Sugars
11.4 g Protein

Ingredients:

1/2 cup blackberry
1 cup skim milk
1/2 banana, medium
1 tbsp. sugar or honey
1/2 cup ice, crushed

Directions:

1. Add everything to a high speed blender and blend on high settings until smooth & creamy.
2. Add more milk or ice if it looks too thick.
3. Pour the mixture to a tall glass. Serve & enjoy!

Smoothie 11

Strawberry Grapefruit Smoothie

Total preparation & making time: 05 Minutes
Servings: 1

Nutrition Info (Estimated Amount Per Serving)

154 Calories
5 Calories from Fat
0.6 g Total Fat
0.1 g Saturated Fat
0 mg Cholesterol
6.3 mg Sodium
38.9 g Total Carbohydrate
3.9 g Dietary Fiber
11.8 g Sugars
2.8 g Protein

Ingredients:
- 5 strawberries, fresh
- Juice of 1 grapefruit
- 1/2 papaya, medium
- 1/4 cup ice, crushed

Directions:
1. Add everything to a high speed blender and blend on high settings until smooth & creamy.

2. Pour the mixture to a tall glass, preferably chilled. Serve & enjoy!

Smoothie 12

Healthy Smoothie

Total preparation & making time: 05 Minutes
Servings: 2

Nutrition Info (Estimated Amount Per Serving)

97.9 Calories
3 Calories from Fat
0.4 g Total Fat
0.1 g Saturated Fat
0 mg Cholesterol
191.1 mg Sodium
24.8 g Total Carbohydrate
2.2 g Dietary Fiber
21.6 g Sugars
1.4 g Protein

Ingredients:

- 2 and 1/2 cups honeydew melon, diced
- 1 tbsp. lime juice, fresh
- 1/3 cup ginger ale
- 2 tbsp. mint, fresh & chopped
- 6 ice cubes, large

- 1/8 tsp. salt

Directions:

1. Put everything to a high speed blender and blend on high settings until smooth & creamy.

Smoothie 13

Strawberry Apple Smoothie

Total preparation & making time: 05 Minutes
Servings: 2

Nutrition Info (Estimated Amount Per Serving)

206.5 Calories
24 Calories from Fat
2.7 g Total Fat
1 g Saturated Fat
6.5 mg Cholesterol
68.5 mg Sodium
42.9 g Total Carbohydrate
5.2 g Dietary Fiber
23.4 g Sugars
6 g Protein

Ingredients:
- 1/2 cup milk, 1% low-fat
- 1/2 cup strawberry yogurt or vanilla yogurt or any of your favorite fruit yogurt
- 2 tsp. honey
- 1 cup strawberries, frozen
- 1 apple, peeled & cored
- 2 tsp. flax seeds, ground

Directions:

1. Add everything together in a high speed blender; whirl on high settings until smooth.
2. Add a dollop of whipping cream over the top, if you want your smoothie to look like more of a dessert.

Smoothie 14

Strawberry Smoothie

Total preparation & making time: 05 Minutes
Servings: 4

Nutrition Info (Estimated Amount Per Serving)

111.5 Calories
2 Calories from Fat
0.3 g Total Fat
0 g Saturated Fat
0 mg Cholesterol
3.5 mg Sodium
28.4 g Total Carbohydrate
1.5 g Dietary Fiber
25.5 g Sugars
0.6 g Protein

Ingredients:

- 2 cups chilled strawberries
- 0.5 can lemonade concentrate, frozen (6 oz.)
- 2 and 1/2 cups ice cubes, small or crushed ice
- 1/3 cup sifted sugar, powdered

Directions:

1. Add the lemon concentrate to a high speed blender; add in the powdered sugar & strawberries.
2. Finally add in the ice cubes. Cover & blend on high settings until nearly smooth.

Smoothie 15

Pumpkin Smoothie

Total preparation & making time: 05 Minutes
Servings: 2

Nutrition Info (Estimated Amount Per Serving)

55.5 Calories
4 Calories from Fat
0.5 g Total Fat
0.2 g Saturated Fat
0 mg Cholesterol
303.5 mg Sodium
13.2 g Total Carbohydrate
3.7 g Dietary Fiber
6.5 g Sugars
1.5 g Protein

Ingredients:

- 1/2 cup pumpkin, canned & not pumpkin pie mix
- 3 packets sugar substitute, (1 g)
- 1/2 tsp. pumpkin spice
- 6 to 8 ice cubes
- 1/2 cup soymilk, low-fat or reduced-fat milk
- 1 tbsp. hot water
- 1/2 cup water, cold

Directions:

1. Put your favorite sweetener in one tbsp. of hot water; stir well until completely dissolved.
2. Add everything together (except the ice) to a high speed blender.
3. Whiz couple of times & then add in the ice. Cover & blend on high setting until ice is crushed completely & the mixture is smooth.

Smoothie 16

Apple Pie Smoothie

Total preparation & making time: 05 Minutes
Servings: 2

Nutrition Info (Estimated Amount Per Serving)

96.4 Calories
19 Calories from Fat
2.1 g Total Fat
1.3 g Saturated Fat
8 mg Cholesterol
32 mg Sodium
17.6 g Total Carbohydrate
0.3 g Dietary Fiber
16.4 g Sugars
2.2 g Protein

Ingredients:
- 1/2 cup vanilla yogurt
- 1 cup apple juice
- 1/4 tsp. cinnamon

Directions:
1. Add everything to a high speed blender and blend on high settings until smooth & creamy.

2. Pour the mixture to tall glasses, preferably chilled. Serve & enjoy!

Smoothie 17

Cucumber Honeydew Smoothies

Total preparation & making time: 05 Minutes
Servings: 2

Nutrition Info (Estimated Amount Per Serving)

36.1 Calories
1 Calories from Fat
0.1 g Total Fat
0 g Saturated Fat
0 mg Cholesterol
94 mg Sodium
9.1 g Total Carbohydrate
0.8 g Dietary Fiber
7.6 g Sugars
0.7 g Protein

Ingredients:

- 1 cup honeydew melon, chopped & chilled
- 1/2 cup cucumber, peeled, seeded, chopped & chilled
- Cucumbers, slices or lime wedges or honeydew melon, chunks
- 1/2 tsp. lime juice
- 1 dash salt

Directions:

1. Add honeydew melon together with the cucumber, lime juice, & salt to a high speed blender. Cover and blend on high settings until smooth & creamy.
2. Garnish each serving with lime wedges and honeydew melon chunks and/or cucumber slices threaded onto skewer

Smoothie 18

Cranberry Orange Smoothie

Total preparation & making time: 05 Minutes
Servings: 1

Nutrition Info (Estimated Amount Per Serving)

80.1 Calories
2 Calories from Fat
0.2 g Total Fat
0 g Saturated Fat
0 mg Cholesterol
7.5 mg Sodium
20.6 g Total Carbohydrate
4.2 g Dietary Fiber
12.9 g Sugars
1.4 g Protein

Ingredients:

- 1 navel orange, large, peeled & break in half
- 1/4 cup cranberries, fresh
- 6 ice cubes
- 1/4 cup water

Directions:

1. Add everything to a high speed blender and blend on high settings until smooth & creamy.
2. Pour the mixture to a tall glass. Serve & enjoy!

Smoothie 19

Spinach Smoothie

Total preparation & making time: 15 Minutes
Servings: 2

Nutrition Info (Estimated Amount Per Serving)

156.7 Calories
7 Calories from Fat
0.9 g Total Fat
0.2 g Saturated Fat
0 mg Cholesterol
91.7 mg Sodium
37.9 g Total Carbohydrate
7.8 g Dietary Fiber
23.3 g Sugars
4.7 g Protein

Ingredients:
- 1 apple, peeled & sliced (Granny Smith or Golden Delicious)
- 1 banana, medium, frozen, peeled & sliced
- 8 oz. Spinach or Kale or Arugula, fresh
- 1 orange, peeled
- Maple syrup or your favorite sweetener to taste

- 1 cup water

Directions:
1. Add everything to a high speed blender and blend on high settings until smooth & creamy. Taste and adjust the level of sweetener, if desired.
2. Pour the mixture to tall glasses, preferably chilled. Serve & enjoy!

Smoothie 20

Berries Pineapple Smoothie

Total preparation & making time: 05 Minutes
Servings: 4

Nutrition Info (Estimated Amount Per Serving)

149.3 Calories
2 Calories from Fat
0.3 g Total Fat
0 g Saturated Fat
0 mg Cholesterol
10.6 mg Sodium
38.4 g Total Carbohydrate
6.7 g Dietary Fiber
28 g Sugars
1.4 g Protein

Ingredients:

- 1 and 1/2 cups strawberries, frozen
- 1 cup raspberries, frozen
- 355 ml diet Sprite
- 1 cup pineapple, chopped into small pieces

Directions:

1. Add everything to a high speed blender and blend on high settings until smooth & creamy.
2. Pour the mixture to glasses, preferably chilled and with straws or spoons. Serve & enjoy!

Smoothie 21

Carrot Mango Smoothie

Total preparation & making time: 05 Minutes
Servings: 2

Nutrition Info (Estimated Amount Per Serving)

186 Calories
23 Calories from Fat
2.6 g Total Fat
1.4 g Saturated Fat
7.4 mg Cholesterol
47.5 mg Sodium
39.9 g Total Carbohydrate
3.2 g Dietary Fiber
33.5 g Sugars
4 g Protein

Ingredients:
- 2 cups mangoes, frozen & chunks
- 1/2 cup carrot juice
- 4 oz. vanilla yogurt
- 1/2 cup apple juice

Directions:
1. Add everything to a high speed blender and blend on high settings until smooth & creamy.

2. Serve in a fun cup or glass with a straw

Smoothie 22

Orange Melon Smoothies

Total preparation & making time: 05 Minutes
Servings: 4

Nutrition Info (Estimated Amount Per Serving)

144.5 Calories
10 Calories from Fat
1.2 g Total Fat
0.6 g Saturated Fat
3.4 mg Cholesterol
48 mg Sodium
30 g Total Carbohydrate
0.7 g Dietary Fiber
27.4 g Sugars
4.2 g Protein

Ingredients:

- 1 carton yogurt, plain & low-fat (8 oz.)
- 2 cups orange juice, chilled
- 1/2 tsp. vanilla
- 1 cup cantaloupe, cubed & chilled
- 3 tbsp. sugar or honey

- Wheat germ, toasted

Directions:

1. Add everything to a high speed blender. Cover & blend on high settings until smooth & creamy.
2. Garnish with additional cantaloupe and sprinkle each serving with wheat germ, if desired. Serve & enjoy!

Smoothie 23

Green Smoothie

Total preparation & making time: 05 Minutes
Servings: 2

Nutrition Info (Estimated Amount Per Serving)

207 Calories
5 Calories from Fat
0.6 g Total Fat
0.2 g Saturated Fat
2.5 mg Cholesterol
124 mg Sodium
44.4 g Total Carbohydrate
3.2 g Dietary Fiber
36.1 g Sugars
8.9 g Protein

Ingredients:
- 1 to 2 bananas, medium & frozen
- 3/4 cup pineapple chunk, drained
- 1 cup yogurt, plain & nonfat
- 2 cups Baby Spinach
- 1 cup water, filtered

Directions:

1. First of all you need to add pineapple together with 1/3 of the spinach, yogurt, 1/3 of the spinach, bananas, 1/3 of spinach and water to your high speed blender.
2. Cover & blend on high settings until smooth. Serve over ice!

Smoothie 24

Banana Kale Smoothie

Total preparation & making time: 10 Minutes
Servings: 1

Nutrition Info (Estimated Amount Per Serving)

124.6 Calories
12 Calories from Fat
1.4 g Total Fat
0.8 g Saturated Fat
3.9 mg Cholesterol
29.2 mg Sodium
28.4 g Total Carbohydrate
3.1 g Dietary Fiber
15.8 g Sugars
2.3 g Protein

Ingredients:

- 1 banana, medium
- 2 kale leaves, stem removed
- 1/4 cup nondairy liquid coffee creamer, fat-free & hazelnut-flavored
- 2 tbsp. vanilla yogurt
- 1/8 tsp. coconut extract
- 2 cups ice

Directions:

1. Add everything to a high speed blender and blend on high settings until smooth & creamy.
2. Pour the mixture to a tall glass, preferably chilled. Serve & enjoy!

Smoothie 25

Strawberry Watermelon Smoothie

Total preparation & making time: 05 Minutes
Servings: 4

Nutrition Info (Estimated Amount Per Serving)

105.5 Calories
1 Calories from Fat
0.2 g Total Fat
0 g Saturated Fat
0 mg Cholesterol
3.6 mg Sodium
27.2 g Total Carbohydrate
1.8 g Dietary Fiber
23.1 g Sugars
0.6 g Protein

Ingredients:

- 1 cup watermelon, frozen and into pieces
- 1/4 cup sugar, turbinado
- 1 cup purified water, fresh
- 1/4 tsp. vitamin C powder
- 1 cup strawberries, frozen

Directions:

1. Add everything to a high speed blender and blend on high settings until smooth & creamy.
2. Pour the mixture to glasses, preferably chilled. Serve & enjoy!

Smoothie 26

Minty Green Smoothie

Total preparation & making time: 05 Minutes
Servings: 2

Nutrition Info (Estimated Amount Per Serving)

45.8 Calories
2 Calories from Fat
0.3 g Total Fat
0.1 g Saturated Fat
0 mg Cholesterol
29 mg Sodium
11.1 g Total Carbohydrate
1.4 g Dietary Fiber
7.6 g Sugars
1.6 g Protein

Ingredients:

- 2 cups spinach, raw
- 1/2 cup grapes, white or green
- 8 mint sprigs, fresh and to taste
- 1/2 cucumber, peeled
- 3 to 4 ice cubes
- 1 cup water

Directions:

1. Add everything to a high speed blender and blend on high settings until smooth & creamy.
2. Pour the mixture to a tall glass, preferably chilled. Serve & enjoy!

Smoothie 27

Salad Smoothie

Total preparation & making time: 10 Minutes
Servings: 1

Nutrition Info (Estimated Amount Per Serving)

99.7 Calories
7 Calories from Fat
0.8 g Total Fat
0.2 g Saturated Fat
0 mg Cholesterol
665.8 mg Sodium
22.4 g Total Carbohydrate
6.3 g Dietary Fiber
10.8 g Sugars
4.8 g Protein

Ingredients:

- 4 to 6 lettuce leaves (Bibb, romaine or a mix)
- 1 carrot, peeled
- 1/2 cucumber, peeled
- 8 cherry tomatoes, stemmed
- 1 scallion, trimmed
- 1/2 tsp. lemon juice, fresh
- 1/4 tsp. salt

- 1 cherry tomatoes, for garnish
- 1 whole scallion, for garnish

Directions:

1. Wash, trim and chop all the ingredients roughly except the ones for garnish.
2. Blend in a high speed blender until smooth & creamy, preferably on high settings.
3. Pour into glass; garnish with cherry tomato & scallion stirrer.

Thank You

Before you go, I'd like to say "thank you" again for purchasing my book. I hope you enjoyed reading the book and you'll try all these smoothies. I know you could have picked from dozens of books on weight loss smoothies, but you took a chance with my book and that means everything to me. So a BIG THANKS for downloading this book and reading all the way to the end. Now I'd like ask for a "SMALL" favor. Please take a minute or two and leave a review for my book.

Thank you again!

Linda